CANDIDA DIET FOOD LIST

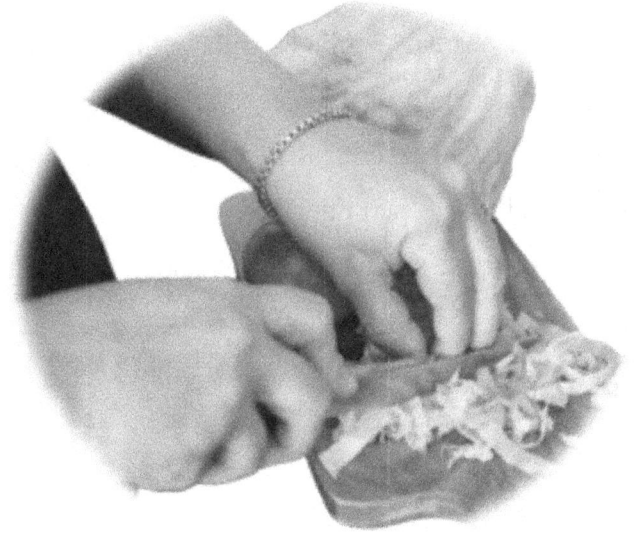

THE ULTIMATE GUIDE TO DIETARY FOODS WITH 28 DELICIOUS AND NUTRITIOUS RECIPES TO FIGHT YEAST AND BEAT CANDIDA FOR YOUR OVERALL WELL-BEING.

Dr. Fiona Henry

ADDITIONAL TITLES BY THIS AUTHOR

- ❖ *The Complete Iron Deficiency Anemia Cookbook*
- ❖ *Mediterranean Diet Cookbook for Iron Deficiency Anemia*
- ❖ *Osteoarthritis Diet Cookbook for Seniors*
- ❖ *Mediterranean Diet Cookbook for Osteoarthritis*
- ❖ *Mediterranean Diet Cookbook for Rheumatoid Arthritis*

SCAN THE QR-CODE BELOW

EXTRA BONUS

BONUS

WEEKLY MEAL PLANNER

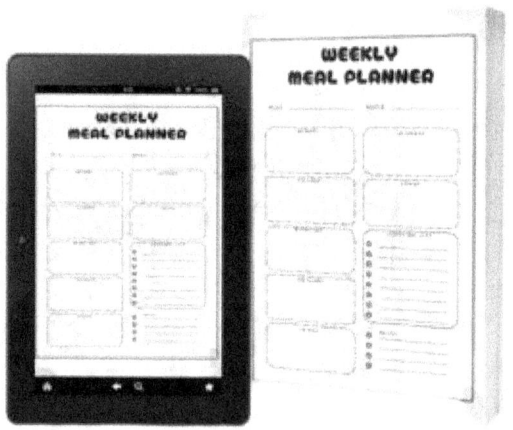

TABLE OF CONTENTS

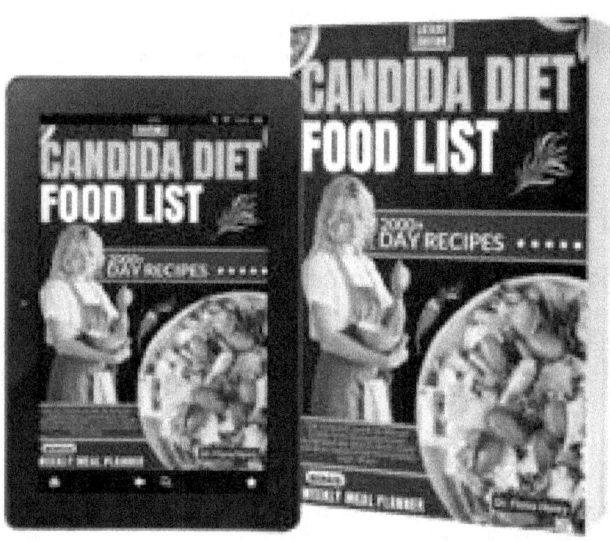

INTRODUCTION

Greetings, dear readers, and welcome to the enlightening journey that lies ahead within the pages of "Candida Diet Food List: The Ultimate Guide to Dietary Foods with 28 Delicious and Nutritious Recipes to Fight Yeast and Beat Candida for Your Overall Well-Being." It is my distinct pleasure to extend my hand in guidance through this labyrinth of nutrition, as Dr. Fiona Henry, a stalwart practitioner in the realm of dietary wellness.

Allow me to introduce myself, for our paths may not have crossed before. I am Dr. Fiona Henry, a seasoned doctor in nutrition with a passion for empowering individuals to take control of their health through mindful eating and informed dietary choices. With years of experience under my belt and a fervent dedication to the well-being of my patients, I have witnessed the transformative power of nutrition in shaping lives and restoring vitality.

Throughout my illustrious career, I have traversed the vast landscape of nutritional science, delving deep into its mysteries and emerging armed with knowledge to guide those in need.

From bustling clinics to serene counseling sessions, I have lent my expertise to individuals from all walks of life, offering solace and support in their quest for wellness.

Now, let us turn our attention to the enigmatic phenomenon known as Candida overgrowth, a topic that has perplexed many and eluded understanding for far too long. Candida overgrowth, characterized by an imbalance of the naturally occurring yeast Candida albicans in the body, is a condition that affects millions worldwide, yet often remains shrouded in mystery.

Picture this: within the intricate ecosystem of the human body, Candida albicans, a microscopic organism, exists in harmony with other microorganisms, contributing to the delicate balance of our internal milieu. However, when this equilibrium is disrupted, be it by antibiotic use, dietary imbalances, or weakened immunity, Candida albicans can seize the opportunity to proliferate unchecked, wreaking havoc on our health in the process.

The manifestations of Candida overgrowth are as varied as they are insidious, ranging from digestive disturbances and skin ailments to chronic fatigue and mood disorders.

Indeed, the symptoms of Candida overgrowth can masquerade as a multitude of other conditions, confounding both patients and healthcare practitioners alike.

But fear not, for within the pages of this guide lies the key to unraveling the mysteries of Candida overgrowth and reclaiming control of your health. Together, we shall embark on a journey of discovery, exploring the signs and symptoms, unraveling the underlying causes and risk factors, and illuminating the path to prevention and treatment.

As we navigate the labyrinthine corridors of Candida overgrowth, I shall be your steadfast companion, guiding you with wisdom garnered from years of experience and a deep-seated passion for nutritional healing. Together, we shall unlock the secrets of the Candida diet, an approach that seeks to starve the yeast by eliminating its favorite foods while nourishing the body with wholesome, Candida-friendly alternatives.

But our journey does not end there, for nestled within these pages lie a treasure trove of delectable recipes designed to tantalize the taste buds and nourish the body.

From hearty breakfasts to satisfying dinners and refreshing beverages, each recipe is crafted with care to support your journey to wellness.

Thus, I cordially encourage you to embark with me on this life-changing adventure, a voyage of self-awareness, recovery, and empowerment. Together, let us harness the power of nutrition to conquer Candida overgrowth and embark on a path to radiant health and vitality.

The adventure awaits, shall we begin?

What is Candida Overgrowth?

Candida overgrowth, also known as candidiasis, is a condition caused by an imbalance in the naturally occurring yeast Candida albicans in the body. Candida albicans is a type of fungus that resides in various parts of the body, including the mouth, gut, and reproductive organs. Under normal circumstances, Candida albicans coexists harmoniously with other microorganisms, contributing to the body's overall microbial balance. However, when this balance is disrupted, often due to factors such as antibiotic use, dietary imbalances, or compromised immunity, Candida albicans can proliferate unchecked, leading to an overgrowth of yeast.

Signs and Symptoms of Candida Overgrowth:

The signs and symptoms of Candida overgrowth can vary widely, ranging from mild discomfort to debilitating conditions.

Common symptoms may include:

Digestive Issues: Individuals with Candida overgrowth often experience digestive disturbances such as bloating, gas, abdominal pain, diarrhea, or constipation.

Oral Thrush: Candida overgrowth in the mouth can manifest as white patches on the tongue, inner cheeks, or throat, accompanied by discomfort or difficulty swallowing.

Skin Problems: Candida overgrowth may contribute to skin issues such as rashes, itching, redness, or fungal infections like athlete's foot or nail fungus.

Fatigue and Weakness: Chronic fatigue and feelings of lethargy are common complaints among individuals with Candida overgrowth, often accompanied by brain fog or difficulty concentrating.

Recurrent Infections: Those with compromised immunity due to Candida overgrowth may experience frequent or recurrent infections, such as urinary tract infections, vaginal yeast infections, or sinus infections.

Mood Disorders: Candida overgrowth has been linked to mood disorders such as depression, anxiety, irritability, or mood swings.

Causes and Risk Factors:

Candida overgrowth can arise due to a number of circumstances, including:

Antibiotic Use: Antibiotics, while effective at treating bacterial infections, can also disrupt the balance of microorganisms in the body, allowing Candida albicans to proliferate.

Dietary Imbalances: Diets high in refined sugars, carbohydrates, and processed foods can fuel the growth of Candida albicans, promoting overgrowth.

Weakened Immunity: Conditions that compromise the immune system, such as HIV/AIDS, autoimmune diseases, or prolonged stress, can increase the risk of Candida overgrowth.

Hormonal Changes: Fluctuations in hormone levels, such as those seen during pregnancy, menstruation, or hormonal therapy, may predispose individuals to Candida overgrowth.

Chronic Illness: Underlying medical conditions such as diabetes, inflammatory bowel disease, or cancer can create an environment conducive to Candida overgrowth.

Preventive Measures:

Preventing Candida overgrowth requires a multifaceted approach aimed at restoring balance to the body's microbiome and addressing underlying risk factors. Some preventive measures include:

Dietary Modifications: Adopting a balanced diet rich in whole foods, fiber, and probiotics while limiting refined sugars, carbohydrates, and processed foods can help maintain a healthy microbial balance and prevent Candida overgrowth.

Probiotic Supplementation: Incorporating probiotic-rich foods or supplements into your diet can support a healthy gut microbiome and inhibit the growth of Candida albicans.

Avoiding Antibiotic Overuse: Whenever possible, avoid unnecessary or prolonged antibiotic use, as this can disrupt the balance of microorganisms in the body and increase the risk of Candida overgrowth.

Managing Stress: Practicing stress-reducing techniques such as mindfulness, meditation, or yoga can help support immune function and reduce the risk of Candida overgrowth.

Maintaining Good Hygiene: Practicing good hygiene, such as regularly washing hands and genital areas, can help prevent the spread of Candida albicans and reduce the risk of infections.

Candida overgrowth is a complex condition characterized by an imbalance of the naturally occurring yeast Candida albicans in the body. Understanding the signs, symptoms, causes, and preventive measures associated with Candida overgrowth is crucial for maintaining optimal health and well-being. By adopting a holistic approach that addresses dietary habits, immune function, and lifestyle factors, you can take proactive steps to prevent Candida overgrowth and promote overall wellness.

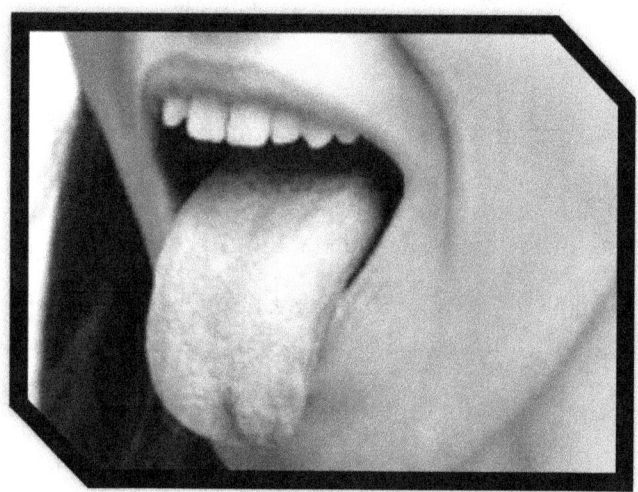

As we journey deeper into the realm of combating Candida overgrowth, it becomes imperative to understand the pivotal role that diet plays in restoring balance to the body's microbial ecosystem. The Candida diet, a cornerstone of our approach in this comprehensive guide, is a strategic dietary protocol designed to starve the yeast while nourishing the body with wholesome, Candida-friendly alternatives. Let us unravel the intricacies of this transformative dietary approach and equip ourselves with the knowledge needed to embark on a path to wellness.

Foods to Avoid on the Candida Diet:

To effectively combat Candida overgrowth, it is essential to eliminate or significantly reduce certain foods that fuel the growth of yeast and exacerbate symptoms. These include:

Sugars and Sweeteners: Refined sugars, high-fructose corn syrup, and artificial sweeteners provide fuel for Candida albicans, promoting its proliferation. Steer clear of sugary treats, sodas, candies, and desserts to starve the yeast and hinder its growth.

Carbohydrates: Simple carbohydrates such as white bread, pasta, rice, and baked goods can quickly break down into sugars in the body, feeding Candida overgrowth. Opt for complex carbohydrates found in whole grains, vegetables, and legumes to provide sustained energy without fueling the yeast.

Processed Foods: Processed foods often contain additives, preservatives, and hidden sugars that can disrupt the body's microbial balance and exacerbate Candida overgrowth. Choose whole, unprocessed foods whenever possible to support optimal health and well-being.

Dairy Products: Dairy products, particularly those high in lactose, can contribute to inflammation and promote the growth of Candida albicans. Consider alternatives such as almond milk, coconut milk, or dairy-free cheeses to support your Candida diet journey.

Alcohol: Alcohol not only disrupts the body's microbial balance but also weakens the immune system, making it more susceptible to Candida overgrowth. Limit or avoid alcohol consumption to optimize your body's ability to combat yeast overgrowth.

Foods to Enjoy on the Candida Diet:

While certain foods may exacerbate Candida overgrowth, others can help support your body's natural defenses and promote a healthy microbial balance. Incorporate the following Candida-friendly foods into your diet to nourish your body and support your journey to wellness:

Non-Starchy Vegetables: Fill your plate with an array of colorful, non-starchy vegetables such as leafy greens, cruciferous vegetables, peppers, and mushrooms. These nutrient-dense foods provide essential vitamins, minerals, and antioxidants to support immune function and combat Candida overgrowth.

Lean Proteins: Choose lean sources of protein such as poultry, fish, eggs, and plant-based proteins like tofu, tempeh, and legumes. Protein is essential for supporting muscle growth and repair while helping to stabilize blood sugar levels and reduce cravings for sugary foods.

Healthy Fats: Incorporate healthy fats such as avocados, nuts, seeds, and olive oil into your diet to support brain health, hormone production, and inflammation reduction.

These heart-healthy fats provide sustained energy and satiety without promoting Candida overgrowth.

Fermented Foods: Fermented foods like yogurt, kefir, sauerkraut, and kimchi contain beneficial probiotics that help restore balance to the gut microbiome and inhibit the growth of Candida albicans. Include a variety of fermented foods in your diet to promote digestive health and immune function.

Essential Tips for Success on the Candida Diet:

Consider the following essential tips to support your Candida diet journey and maximize your chances of success:

Be Mindful of Hidden Sugars: Read food labels carefully and be mindful of hidden sugars in processed foods, condiments, sauces, and beverages. Opt for sugar-free or naturally sweetened alternatives to avoid inadvertently fueling Candida overgrowth.

Plan Ahead: Take the time to plan your meals and snacks in advance to ensure that you have healthy, Candida-friendly options on hand. Stock your pantry with nutritious staples and prepare meals in bulk to save time and energy throughout the week.

Stay Hydrated: Drink plenty of water throughout the day to support hydration, detoxification, and digestive health. Herbal teas, infused water, and coconut water are excellent hydrating options that can also help curb cravings and promote satiety.

Practice Self-Care: Prioritize self-care practices such as adequate sleep, stress management, and regular exercise to support your body's natural defenses and promote overall well-being. Engage in activities that bring you joy and relaxation to reduce stress and support your Candida diet journey.

Seek Support: Surround yourself with a supportive community of friends, family, or fellow Candida diet enthusiasts who can offer encouragement, accountability, and guidance along your journey. Share your experiences, challenges, and successes with others to stay motivated and inspired.

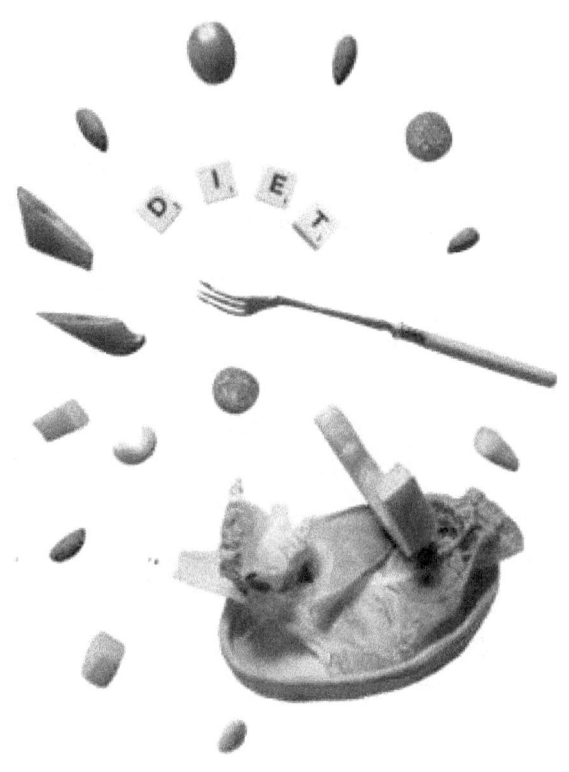

COMPREHENSIVE LIST OF CANDIDA-FRIENDLY FOODS

1. Non-Starchy Vegetables:

Leafy greens such as spinach, kale, collard greens, and Swiss chard are rich in fiber, vitamins, and minerals that support digestive health and immune function.

Cruciferous vegetables like broccoli, cauliflower, and Brussels sprouts contain compounds that support liver detoxification and have anti-inflammatory properties.

Cucumbers, asparagus, zucchini, bell peppers, celery, and green beans are low in sugar and provide essential nutrients without feeding candida.

2. Low-Sugar Fruits (in moderation):

Berries such as blueberries, strawberries, and raspberries are rich in antioxidants and low in sugar, making them suitable choices for a candida diet.

Green apples are lower in sugar compared to other varieties and provide fiber and vitamins.

The fruit avocado is high in nutrients and contains a lot of fiber, potassium, and healthy fats.

3. Protein Sources:

Wild-caught fish like salmon, mackerel, and sardines are excellent sources of omega-3 fatty acids, which have anti-inflammatory properties.

Organic poultry such as chicken and turkey provide lean protein and essential nutrients.

Grass-fed beef is a source of high-quality protein, iron, and zinc.

Eggs, preferably organic and pasture-raised, are rich in protein and essential nutrients.

Plant-based proteins like tofu, tempeh, and legumes (in moderation) provide protein, fiber, and other nutrients essential for overall health.

4. Healthy Fats:

Coconut oil contains caprylic acid, a natural antifungal compound, and medium-chain triglycerides (MCTs) that support energy production and immune function.

Olive oil (extra virgin) is rich in antioxidants and monounsaturated fats that have anti-inflammatory properties.

Avocado oil is a source of monounsaturated fats and vitamin E, which support heart health and immune function.

Flaxseed oil is rich in omega-3 fatty acids, which have anti-inflammatory properties and support brain health.

Nuts and seeds like almonds, walnuts, chia seeds, flaxseeds, hemp seeds, and pumpkin seeds provide healthy fats, protein, fiber, and essential nutrients.

5. Fermented Foods:

Kimchi, a traditional Korean fermented vegetable dish, contains probiotics that support gut health and immune function.

Sauerkraut, made from fermented cabbage, is rich in probiotics and enzymes that aid digestion.

Kombucha, a fermented tea beverage, contains probiotics and antioxidants, but it's important to choose varieties with low sugar content.

Unsweetened coconut yogurt is dairy-free and contains probiotics that support gut health.

Fermented pickles made without added sugar provide probiotics and can be a tasty addition to a candida-friendly diet.

6. Herbs and Spices:

Garlic contains allicin, a compound with potent antimicrobial properties that may help combat candida overgrowth.

Ginger has anti-inflammatory and antioxidant properties and may help support digestion and immune function.

Turmeric contains curcumin, a compound with anti-inflammatory and antioxidant properties that may support immune function and overall health.

Cinnamon has antimicrobial properties and may help regulate blood sugar levels.

Oregano contains carvacrol and thymol, compounds with antifungal properties.

Thyme, basil, rosemary, and parsley are culinary herbs that add flavor to dishes and may have antimicrobial properties.

7. Beverages:

Herbal teas such as peppermint, ginger, and chamomile are caffeine-free and may have digestive benefits.

Green tea, consumed in moderation, contains polyphenols and antioxidants that support overall health.

Water, whether filtered or spring water, is essential for hydration and helps flush toxins from the body.

Unsweetened coconut water is a natural source of electrolytes and may help replenish fluids and minerals.

8. Grains and Alternatives:

Quinoa is a gluten-free pseudo-grain rich in protein, fiber, and essential nutrients.

Buckwheat is a gluten-free grain-like seed that provides protein, fiber, and minerals.

Millet is a gluten-free grain that is easily digestible and provides carbohydrates for energy.

Amaranth is a gluten-free pseudo-grain rich in protein, fiber, and micronutrients.

Brown rice, consumed in moderation, is a whole grain that provides carbohydrates and essential nutrients.

9. Sweeteners:

Stevia is a natural, non-caloric sweetener derived from the leaves of the Stevia rebaudiana plant.

Monk fruit extract, used in moderation, is a natural sweetener derived from the monk fruit that contains antioxidants and has no impact on blood sugar levels.

10. Dairy Alternatives:

Unsweetened almond milk is a dairy-free alternative rich in calcium, vitamin E, and other nutrients.

Coconut milk is a dairy-free alternative rich in medium-chain triglycerides (MCTs) and vitamins.

Cashew milk is a dairy-free alternative that provides protein, healthy fats, and essential nutrients.

Hemp milk is a dairy-free alternative rich in omega-3 fatty acids, protein, and essential nutrients.

11. Other Considerations:

Limit or avoid added sugars, refined carbohydrates, and processed foods, as they can promote candida overgrowth.

Choose organic, non-GMO options whenever possible to minimize exposure to pesticides and toxins.

Stay hydrated by drinking plenty of water throughout the day to support detoxification and overall health.

Consider incorporating anti-fungal supplements or herbs like berberine, caprylic acid, oregano oil, and grapefruit seed extract under the guidance of a healthcare professional.

Practice stress management techniques such as mindfulness, meditation, yoga, or deep breathing exercises, as stress can weaken the immune system and exacerbate candida overgrowth.

Engage in regular physical activity to support circulation, digestion, and overall well-being.

Prioritize adequate sleep to support immune function, hormone regulation, and overall health.

By incorporating the foods listed above into your diet and making lifestyle modifications to support digestive health, immune function, and overall well-being, you can help fight and beat candida overgrowth naturally. It's essential to listen to your body, work with a healthcare professional or registered dietitian, and make dietary changes gradually to achieve long-term success in managing candida overgrowth and promoting optimal health.

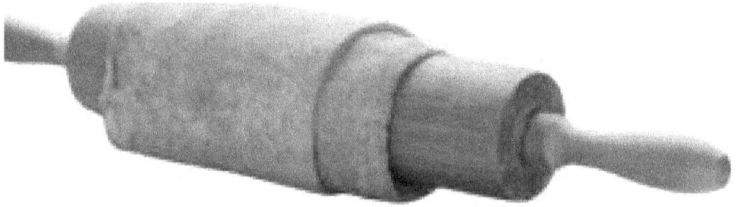

BREAKFAST RECIPES

Coconut Flour Pancakes:

Ingredients:

- 1/4 cup coconut flour
- 2 tablespoons almond flour
- 2 eggs
- 1/4 cup unsweetened almond milk
- 1 tablespoon coconut oil, melted
- 1/2 teaspoon baking powder
- Pinch of salt
- Optional: Stevia or erythritol to taste
- Fresh berries for topping

Preparation:

1. In a mixing bowl, whisk together coconut flour, almond flour, baking powder, and salt.
2. In a separate bowl, beat the eggs, then add almond milk, melted coconut oil, and sweetener (if using).
3. Gradually add the wet ingredients to the dry ingredients, stirring until well combined and smooth.
4. Heat a non-stick skillet over medium heat and lightly grease with coconut oil.
5. Pour small amounts of batter onto the skillet to form pancakes.
6. Fry until surface bubbles appear, then turn and continue cooking until both sides are golden brown.
7. Serve warm with fresh berries on top.

Portion Size: 2-3 pancakes

Cooking Time: 10-15 minutes

Nutritional Information (per serving):

- Calories: 200
- Protein: 9g
- Fat: 12g
- Carbohydrates: 14g
- Fiber: 8g

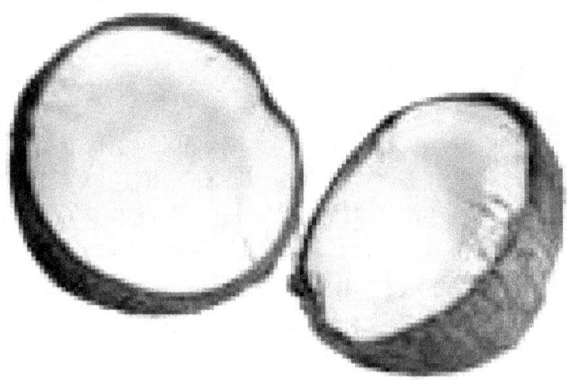

Greek Yogurt Parfait:

Ingredients:

- 1/2 cup plain Greek yogurt
- 1/4 cup mixed berries (such as strawberries, blueberries, raspberries)
- 1 tablespoon almond butter or coconut flakes
- Optional: Stevia or erythritol to taste
- Sprinkle of cinnamon

Preparation:

1. In a serving glass or bowl, layer Greek yogurt, mixed berries, and almond butter or coconut flakes.
2. Sweeten with stevia or erythritol if desired.
3. Sprinkle with cinnamon for added flavor.
4. Repeat layering if desired.
5. Serve chilled or at room temperature.

Portion Size: 1 serving

Preparation Time: 5 minutes

Nutritional Information (per serving):

- Calories: 180
- Protein: 15g
- Fat: 7g
- Carbohydrates: 15g
- Fiber: 5g

Veggie Omelette:

Ingredients:

- 2 eggs
- 2 tablespoons unsweetened almond milk
- 1/4 cup chopped vegetables (such as bell peppers, onions, spinach)
- 1 tablespoon olive oil or coconut oil
- Salt and pepper to taste
- Optional: Fresh herbs for garnish

Preparation:

1. In a bowl, whisk together eggs, almond milk, salt, and pepper until well combined.
2. In a non-stick skillet, heat the oil over medium heat.
3. Add chopped vegetables to the skillet and sauté until tender.
4. Pour the egg mixture over the vegetables in the skillet.
5. Cook until the edges start to set, then gently lift the edges and tilt the skillet to allow the uncooked egg mixture to flow to the bottom.
6. Continue cooking until the omelette is set and lightly golden on the bottom.
7. Fold the omelette in half and transfer to a plate.
8. Garnish with fresh herbs if desired.
9. Serve hot.

Portion Size: 1 omelette

Cooking Time: 10 minutes

Nutritional Information (per serving):

- Calories: 200
- Protein: 12g
- Fat: 15g
- Carbohydrates: 5g
- Fiber: 2g

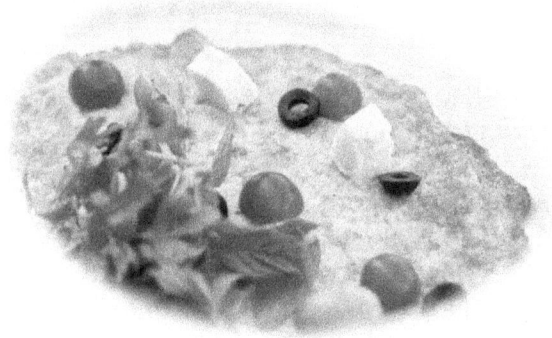

Almond Flour Muffins:

Ingredients:

- 1 cup almond flour
- 1/4 cup coconut flour
- 2 eggs
- 1/4 cup unsweetened almond milk
- 1/4 cup coconut oil, melted
- 1/4 cup raw honey or maple syrup
- 1 teaspoon baking powder
- Pinch of salt
- Optional: Berries or chopped nuts for added flavor

Preparation:

1. Preheat the oven to 350°F (175°C) and line a muffin tin with paper liners.
2. Combine almond flour, coconut flour, baking powder, and salt in a mixing dish.
3. In a separate bowl, whisk together eggs, almond milk, melted coconut oil, and sweetener.
4. Stirring until thoroughly blended, gradually add the wet components to the dry ingredients.
5. Fold in berries or chopped nuts if desired.
6. Spoon the batter into the prepared muffin tin, filling each cup about 2/3 full.
7. Bake for 20-25 minutes, or until golden brown and a toothpick inserted into the center comes out clean.
8. Allow the muffins to cool in the tin for 5 minutes, then transfer to a wire rack to cool completely.
9. Serve warm or at room temperature.

Portion Size: 1 muffin

Cooking Time: 25 minutes

Nutritional Information (per serving):

- Calories: 180
- Protein: 5g
- Fat: 12g
- Carbohydrates: 15g
- Fiber: 3g

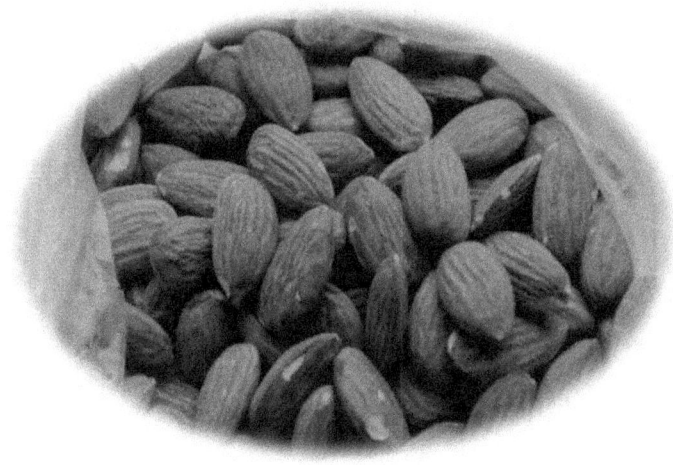

Green Smoothie Bowl:

Ingredients:

- 1 cup spinach or kale
- 1/2 frozen banana
- 1/4 avocado
- 1/2 cup unsweetened almond milk or coconut water
- 1 tablespoon chia seeds
- Optional toppings: sliced strawberries, shredded coconut, granola

Preparation:

1. In a blender, combine spinach or kale, frozen banana, avocado, almond milk or coconut water, and chia seeds.
2. Blend until smooth and creamy.
3. Pour the smoothie into a bowl and top with sliced strawberries, shredded coconut, and granola if desired.
4. Serve immediately with a spoon.

Portion Size: 1 bowl

Preparation Time: 5 minutes

Nutritional Information (per serving):

- Calories: 250
- Protein: 7g
- Fat: 12g
- Carbohydrates: 30g
- Fiber: 10g

Quinoa Breakfast Bowl:

Ingredients:

- 1/2 cup cooked quinoa
- 1/4 cup unsweetened almond milk or coconut milk
- 1 tablespoon almond butter or tahini
- 1 tablespoon hemp seeds or flaxseeds
- 1/4 cup of mixed berries, including raspberries and blueberries
- Optional: Cinnamon or nutmeg for flavor

Preparation:

1. In a serving bowl, combine cooked quinoa, almond milk or coconut milk, almond butter or tahini, and hemp seeds or flaxseeds.
2. Stir until well combined and creamy.
3. Top with mixed berries and sprinkle with cinnamon or nutmeg if desired.
4. Serve warm or at room temperature.

Portion Size: 1 serving

Preparation Time: 10 minutes

Nutritional Information (per serving):

- Calories: 300
- Protein: 10g
- Fat: 15g
- Carbohydrates: 30g
- Fiber: 6g

Baked Sweet Potato Breakfast Hash:

Ingredients:

- 1 medium sweet potato, peeled and diced
- 1/2 red bell pepper, diced
- 1/4 red onion, diced
- 2 cloves garlic, minced
- 1 tablespoon coconut oil or olive oil
- Salt and pepper to taste
- 2 eggs
- Optional: Fresh herbs for garnish

Preparation:

1. Preheat the oven to 400°F (200°C).
2. In a baking dish, toss together diced sweet potato, red bell pepper, red onion, minced garlic, coconut oil or olive oil, salt, and pepper.
3. Bake for 25-30 minutes, or until the sweet potatoes are tender and golden brown.
4. Remove from the oven and make two wells in the hash mixture.
5. Crack an egg into each well.
6. Return the baking dish to the oven and bake for an additional 10-12 minutes, or until the eggs are set to your liking.
7. Garnish with fresh herbs if desired.
8. Serve hot.

Portion Size: 1/2 of the hash with 1 egg

Cooking Time: 35-40 minutes

Nutritional Information (per serving):

- Calories: 250
- Protein: 10g
- Fat: 12g
- Carbohydrates: 25g
- Fiber: 5g

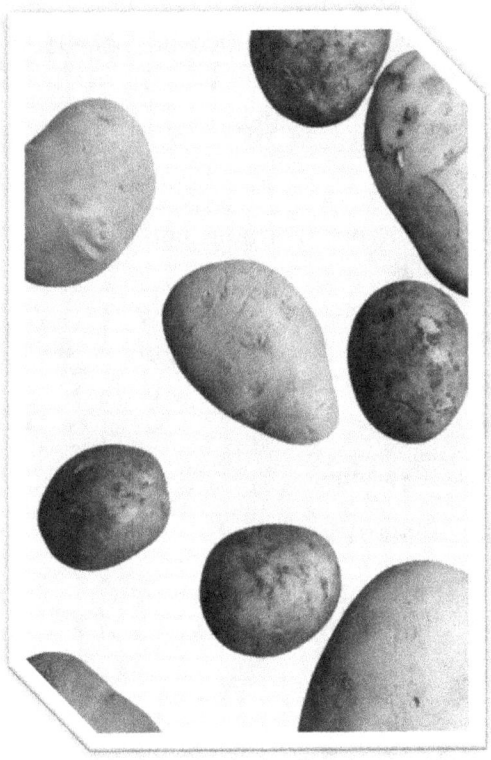

LUNCH RECIPES

Quinoa and Veggie Buddha Bowl:

Ingredients:

- 1/2 cup cooked quinoa
- 1 cup mixed vegetables (such as roasted sweet potatoes, steamed broccoli, sautéed bell peppers)
- 1/4 cup chickpeas, drained and rinsed
- 2 tablespoons hummus
- 1 tablespoon tahini dressing (made with tahini, lemon juice, garlic, and water)
- Fresh herbs for garnish

Preparation:

1. In a serving bowl, arrange cooked quinoa and mixed vegetables.
2. Add chickpeas on top.
3. Drizzle with hummus and tahini dressing.
4. Garnish with fresh herbs.
5. Serve immediately.

Portion Size: 1 serving

Preparation Time: 15 minutes

Nutritional Information (per serving):

- Calories: 350
- Protein: 12g
- Fat: 15g
- Carbohydrates: 45g
- Fiber: 10g

Zucchini Noodles with Avocado Pesto:

Ingredients:

- 2 medium zucchinis, spiralized into noodles
- 1 ripe avocado
- 1/4 cup fresh basil leaves
- 1 clove garlic
- 2 tablespoons lemon juice
- 2 tablespoons olive oil
- Salt and pepper to taste
- Optional: Cherry tomatoes for garnish

Preparation:

1. In a blender or food processor, combine avocado, basil leaves, garlic, lemon juice, olive oil, salt, and pepper. Blend until smooth and creamy.
2. Heat the olive oil in a big skillet over medium heat. Sauté the zucchini noodles until they become soft.
3. Toss the cooked zucchini noodles with avocado pesto until well coated.
4. Garnish with cherry tomatoes if desired.
5. Serve warm or at room temperature.

Portion Size: 1 serving

Cooking Time: 10 minutes

Nutritional Information (per serving):

- Calories: 300
- Protein: 5g
- Fat: 25g
- Carbohydrates: 20g
- Fiber: 10g

Salmon Salad with Lemon Dill Dressing:

Ingredients:

- 1 cup mixed greens
- 4 ounces cooked salmon, flaked
- 1/4 cup cucumber, sliced
- 1/4 cup cherry tomatoes, halved
- 2 tablespoons sliced red onion
- For the dressing: 1 tablespoon olive oil, 1 tablespoon lemon juice, 1 teaspoon chopped fresh dill, salt, and pepper to taste

Preparation:

1. In a large bowl, combine mixed greens, flaked salmon, cucumber slices, cherry tomatoes, and sliced red onion.
2. In a small bowl, whisk together olive oil, lemon juice, chopped fresh dill, salt, and pepper to make the dressing.
3. Drizzle the dressing over the salad and toss until well coated.
4. Serve immediately.

Portion Size: 1 serving

Preparation Time: 10 minutes

Nutritional Information (per serving):

- Calories: 250
- Protein: 20g
- Fat: 15g
- Carbohydrates: 10g
- Fiber: 3g

Cauliflower Fried Rice:

Ingredients:

- 2 cups cauliflower rice
- 1/4 cup mixed vegetables (such as peas, carrots, corn)
- 1/4 cup diced tofu or cooked chicken
- Two tablespoons of coconut aminos or tamari sauce.
- 1 tablespoon sesame oil
- 2 eggs, beaten
- Salt and pepper to taste
- Optional: Chopped green onions for garnish

Preparation:

1. Sesame oil should be heated over medium heat in a large skillet. Add mixed vegetables and diced tofu or cooked chicken. Sauté until vegetables are tender.
2. Push the cooked vegetables to one side of the skillet and add beaten eggs to the other side. Scramble the eggs until cooked through, then combine with the vegetables.
3. Add cauliflower rice and coconut aminos or tamari sauce to the skillet. Stir well to combine.
4. Cook for an additional 3-4 minutes, or until cauliflower rice is heated through.
5. To taste, add salt and pepper for seasoning.
6. If preferred, garnish with finely chopped green onions.
7. Serve hot.

Portion Size: 1 serving

Cooking Time: 15 minutes

Nutritional Information (per serving):

- Calories: 300
- Protein: 15g
- Fat: 15g
- Carbohydrates: 20g
- Fiber: 5g

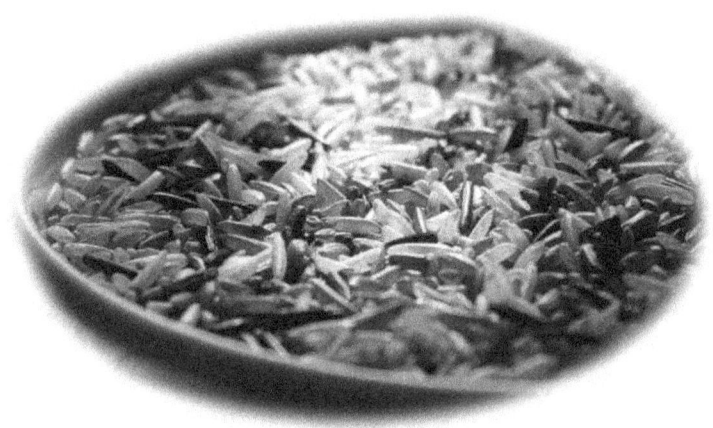

Lentil and Vegetable Soup:

Ingredients:

- 1/2 cup dried lentils
- 2 cups vegetable broth
- 1 cup mixed vegetables (such as carrots, celery, onions)
- 1 clove garlic, minced
- 1 teaspoon dried thyme
- Salt and pepper to taste
- Fresh parsley for garnish

Preparation:

1. In a large pot, combine dried lentils, vegetable broth, mixed vegetables, minced garlic, dried thyme, salt, and pepper.
2. Bring the mixture to a boil, then reduce heat and simmer for 20-25 minutes, or until lentils and vegetables are tender.
3. Adjust seasoning if necessary.
4. Ladle the soup into bowls and garnish with fresh parsley.
5. Serve hot.

Portion Size: 1 serving

Cooking Time: 30 minutes

Nutritional Information (per serving):

- Calories: 250
- Protein: 15g
- Fat: 1g
- Carbohydrates: 45g, Fiber: 15g

Turkey and Avocado Wrap:

Ingredients:

- 1 whole grain or gluten-free wrap
- 3 ounces sliced turkey breast
- 1/4 avocado, mashed
- 1/4 cup mixed greens
- 2 slices tomato
- 1 tablespoon hummus or tahini
- Salt and pepper to taste

Preparation:

1. Lay the wrap flat on a clean surface.
2. Spread mashed avocado evenly over the wrap.
3. Layer sliced turkey breast, mixed greens, tomato slices, and hummus or tahini on top.
4. To taste, add salt and pepper for seasoning.
5. Roll up the wrap tightly.
6. Slice in half if desired.
7. Serve immediately.

Portion Size: 1 wrap

Preparation Time: 5 minutes

Nutritional Information (per serving):

- Calories: 300
- Protein: 20g
- Fat: 15g
- Carbohydrates: 20g
- Fiber: 5g

Chickpea and Vegetable Stir-Fry:

Ingredients:

- 1 cup cooked chickpeas
- One cup of mixed veggies (carrots, snap peas, and bell peppers)
- Two tablespoons of tamari sauce or coconut aminos
- 1 tablespoon sesame oil
- 1 teaspoon grated ginger
- 2 cloves garlic, minced
- Salt and pepper to taste
- Optional: Sliced green onions for garnish

Preparation:

1. Sesame oil should be heated over medium heat in a big skillet. Add mixed vegetables, grated ginger, and minced garlic. Sauté until vegetables are tender.
2. Add cooked chickpeas to the skillet and cook for an additional 2-3 minutes.
3. Stir in coconut aminos or tamari sauce and cook for another 1-2 minutes.
4. Season with salt and pepper to taste.
5. Garnish with sliced green onions if desired.
6. Serve hot over cooked quinoa or brown rice.

Portion Size: 1 serving

Cooking Time: 15 minutes

Nutritional Information (per serving):

- Calories: 300, Protein: 15g
- Fat: 10g
- Carbohydrates: 40g, Fiber: 10g

DINNER RECIPES

Lemon Garlic Baked Salmon:

Ingredients:

- 4 ounces salmon fillet
- 1 tablespoon olive oil
- 1 clove garlic, minced
- 1 tablespoon fresh lemon juice
- 1 teaspoon lemon zest
- Salt and pepper to taste
- Fresh parsley for garnish

Preparation:

1. Before proceeding, preheat the oven to 375°F (190°C) and place parchment paper on a baking pan.
2. Place the salmon fillet on the prepared baking sheet.
3. In a small bowl, whisk together olive oil, minced garlic, lemon juice, lemon zest, salt, and pepper.
4. Pour the lemon garlic mixture over the salmon fillet, ensuring it is evenly coated.
5. Bake for 12-15 minutes, or until the salmon is cooked through and flakes easily with a fork.
6. Garnish with fresh parsley before serving.
7. Serve hot.

Portion Size: 1 serving

Cooking Time: 15 minutes

Nutritional Information (per serving): Calories: 250, Protein: 20g, Fat: 15g, Carbohydrates: 2g

Fiber: 0g

Ingredients:

- 2 cups cauliflower rice
- One cup of mixed veggies, including broccoli, snap peas, and bell peppers
- 1/4 cup cooked shrimp or tofu
- Two tablespoons of tamari sauce or coconut aminos
- 1 tablespoon sesame oil
- 1 teaspoon grated ginger
- 2 cloves garlic, minced
- Salt and pepper to taste
- Optional: Sliced green onions for garnish

Preparation:

1. In a large skillet over medium heat, warm the sesame oil. Add grated ginger and minced garlic, and sauté until fragrant.
2. Add mixed vegetables and cauliflower rice to the skillet. Cook until vegetables are tender.
3. Stir in cooked shrimp or tofu.
4. Add coconut aminos or tamari sauce, and toss until everything is well coated.
5. To taste, add salt and pepper for seasoning.
6. If desired, garnish with chopped green onions.
7. Serve hot.

Portion Size: 1 serving

Cooking Time: 15 minutes

Nutritional Information (per serving): Calories: 200, Protein: 15g, Fat: 10g, Carbohydrates: 15g, Fiber: 7g

Baked Chicken with Roasted Vegetables:

Ingredients:

- 4 ounces chicken breast
- 1 cup mixed vegetables (such as carrots, Brussels sprouts, cauliflower)
- 1 tablespoon olive oil
- 1 teaspoon dried Italian herbs (such as oregano, thyme, basil)
- Salt and pepper to taste
- Fresh parsley for garnish

Preparation:

1. Adjust the oven temperature to 400°F (200°C) and place parchment paper on a baking pan.
2. Place the chicken breast on one side of the prepared baking sheet.
3. Toss mixed vegetables with olive oil, dried Italian herbs, salt, and pepper in a mixing bowl.
4. Arrange the vegetables on the other side of the baking sheet.
5. Bake for 20-25 minutes, or until the chicken is cooked through and the vegetables are tender.
6. Garnish with fresh parsley before serving.
7. Serve hot.

Portion Size: 1 serving

Cooking Time: 25 minutes

Nutritional Information (per serving): Calories: 300, Protein: 25g, Fat: 10g, Carbohydrates: 20g

Turkey and Vegetable Stuffed Bell Peppers:

Ingredients:

- 2 large bell peppers
- 1/2 cup cooked quinoa
- 1/2 cup ground turkey
- 1/4 cup diced tomatoes
- 1/4 cup diced onion
- 1 clove garlic, minced
- 1/4 teaspoon dried oregano
- Salt and pepper to taste
- Optional: Grated cheese for topping

Preparation:

1. Turn the oven on to 375°F (190°C) and coat a baking dish with oil.
2. Slice off the bell peppers' tops, then take out the seeds and membranes.
3. In a skillet, cook ground turkey until browned. Add diced tomatoes, diced onion, minced garlic, dried oregano, salt, and pepper. Cook until vegetables are tender.
4. Stir in cooked quinoa until well combined.
5. Stuff the bell peppers with the turkey and quinoa mixture.
6. Fill the baking dish with the stuffed bell peppers.
7. If desired, top with grated cheese.
8. Bake the bell peppers for 25 to 30 minutes, or until they are soft.
9. Serve hot.

Portion Size: 1 serving

Cooking Time: 30 minutes

Nutritional Information (per serving):

- Calories: 250
- Protein: 20g
- Fat: 10g
- Carbohydrates: 20g
- Fiber: 5g

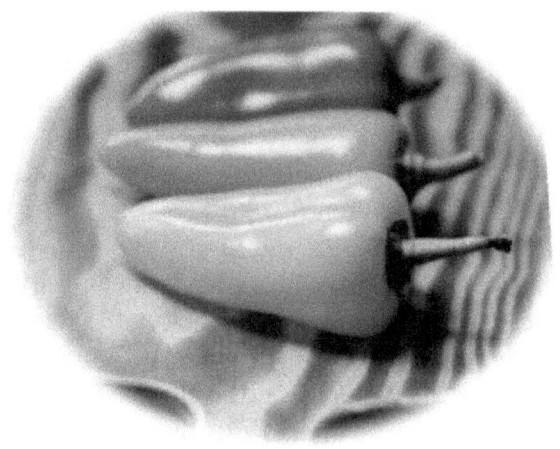

Lentil and Vegetable Curry:

Ingredients:

- 1/2 cup dried lentils
- 2 cups vegetable broth
- 1 cup mixed vegetables (such as carrots, potatoes, peas)
- 1/4 cup coconut milk
- 1 tablespoon curry powder
- 1 clove garlic, minced
- Salt and pepper to taste
- Fresh cilantro for garnish

Preparation:

1. In a large pot, combine dried lentils, vegetable broth, mixed vegetables, coconut milk, curry powder, minced garlic, salt, and pepper.
2. Bring the mixture to a boil, then reduce heat and simmer for 20-25 minutes, or until lentils and vegetables are tender.
3. Adjust seasoning if necessary.
4. Ladle the curry into bowls and garnish with fresh cilantro.
5. Serve hot with cooked quinoa or brown rice.

Portion Size: 1 serving

Cooking Time: 30 minutes

Nutritional Information (per serving): Calories: 300, Protein: 15g, Fat: 10g, Carbohydrates: 40g, Fiber: 15g

Grilled Lemon Herb Chicken with Roasted Asparagus:

Ingredients:

- 4 ounces chicken breast
- 1 tablespoon olive oil
- 1 tablespoon fresh lemon juice
- 1 teaspoon dried Italian herbs (such as rosemary, thyme, parsley)
- Salt and pepper to taste
- 1 bunch asparagus, trimmed
- Optional: Lemon wedges for garnish

Preparation:

1. Preheat the grill to medium-high heat.
2. In a small bowl, whisk together olive oil, lemon juice, dried Italian herbs, salt, and pepper.
3. Brush the chicken breast and asparagus with the lemon herb mixture.
4. Grill the chicken breast for 6-8 minutes per side, or until cooked through.
5. Grill the asparagus for 4-5 minutes, or until tender and slightly charred.
6. Remove the chicken and asparagus from the grill.
7. Garnish with lemon wedges if desired.
8. Serve hot.

Portion Size: 1 serving

Cooking Time: 15 minutes

Nutritional Information (per serving): Calories: 250, Protein: 25g, Fat: 10g, Carbohydrates: 10g, Fiber: 5g

Eggplant and Zucchini Lasagna:

Ingredients:

- 1 large eggplant, sliced lengthwise
- 1 large zucchini, sliced lengthwise
- 1 cup marinara sauce
- 1 cup ricotta cheese
- 1/2 cup shredded mozzarella cheese
- 1/4 cup grated Parmesan cheese
- 1 teaspoon dried Italian herbs
- Salt and pepper to taste
- Fresh basil for garnish

Preparation:

1. Turn the oven on to 375°F (190°C) and coat a baking dish with oil.
2. Spread a thin layer of marinara sauce on the bottom of the baking dish.
3. Arrange sliced eggplant and zucchini in a single layer on top of the marinara sauce.
4. Spread half of the ricotta cheese over the vegetables.
5. Sprinkle with half of the shredded mozzarella cheese and grated Parmesan cheese.
6. Repeat the layers with the remaining vegetables, ricotta cheese, mozzarella cheese, and Parmesan cheese.
7. Sprinkle dried Italian herbs, salt, and pepper on top.
8. Cover the baking dish with foil and bake for 30 minutes.
9. Remove the foil and bake for an additional 15 minutes, or until the cheese is melted and bubbly.
10. Garnish with fresh basil before serving.

11. Allow to cool for a few minutes, then cut into slices and serve.

Portion Size: 1 serving

Cooking Time: 45 minutes

Nutritional Information (per serving):

- Calories: 300
- Protein: 20g
- Fat: 15g
- Carbohydrates: 20g
- Fiber: 7g

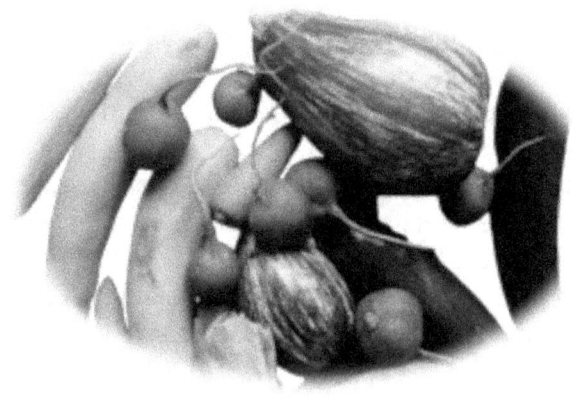

Cucumber Lemon Detox Water:

Ingredients:

- 1 medium cucumber, thinly sliced
- 1 lemon, thinly sliced
- 4 cups filtered water
- Ice cubes (optional)

Preparation:

1. In a large pitcher, combine cucumber and lemon slices.
2. Add filtered water and stir gently to mix.
3. Refrigerate for at least 2 hours to allow flavors to infuse.
4. Serve chilled over ice cubes if desired.

Portion Size: 1 serving

Preparation Time: 5 minutes (plus chilling time)

Nutritional Information (per serving):

- Calories: 0
- Protein: 0g
- Fat: 0g
- Carbohydrates: 0g
- Fiber: 0g

Coconut Berry Smoothie:

Ingredients:

- 1/2 cup mixed berries (such as strawberries, blueberries, raspberries)
- 1/2 cup unsweetened coconut milk
- 1/2 cup plain Greek yogurt (or coconut yogurt for dairy-free option)
- 1 tablespoon chia seeds
- Ice cubes (optional)

Preparation:

1. In a blender, combine mixed berries, coconut milk, Greek yogurt, and chia seeds.
2. Blend until smooth and creamy.
3. Add ice cubes if desired and blend again until well mixed.
4. Pour into a glass and serve immediately.

Portion Size: 1 serving

Preparation Time: 5 minutes

Nutritional Information (per serving):

- Calories: 150
- Protein: 8g
- Fat: 8g
- Carbohydrates: 12g
- Fiber: 6g

Turmeric Ginger Tea:

Ingredients:

- 1 teaspoon ground turmeric
- 1 teaspoon grated ginger
- 2 cups hot water
- 1 tablespoon raw honey (optional)
- Lemon slices for garnish

Preparation:

1. In a mug, add ground turmeric and grated ginger.
2. Pour hot water over the spices and stir well.
3. Allow the tea to steep for 5-10 minutes to infuse flavors.
4. Optionally, add raw honey for sweetness and stir until dissolved.
5. Serve hot, garnished with slices of lemon.

Portion Size: 1 serving

Preparation Time: 10 minutes

Nutritional Information (per serving):

- Calories: 15
- Protein: 0g
- Fat: 0g
- Carbohydrates: 4g
- Fiber: 1g

Green Goddess Smoothie:

Ingredients:

- 1 cup spinach leaves
- 1/2 ripe avocado
- 1/2 cucumber, chopped
- 1/2 cup unsweetened almond milk
- 1 tablespoon fresh lemon juice
- Ice cubes (optional)

Preparation:

1. In a blender, combine spinach leaves, avocado, cucumber, almond milk, and lemon juice.
2. Blend until smooth and creamy.
3. If desired, add ice cubes and blend once more until well combined.
4. Pour into a glass and serve immediately.

Portion Size: 1 serving

Preparation Time: 5 minutes

Nutritional Information (per serving):

- Calories: 150
- Protein: 4g
- Fat: 10g
- Carbohydrates: 12g
- Fiber: 7g

Hibiscus Iced Tea:

Ingredients:

- 2 hibiscus tea bags
- 4 cups boiling water
- 1 tablespoon raw honey (optional)
- Fresh mint leaves for garnish

Preparation:

1. Place hibiscus tea bags in a heatproof pitcher.
2. Pour boiling water over the tea bags and steep for 5-10 minutes.
3. Remove the tea bags and discard.
4. Optionally, add raw honey for sweetness and stir until dissolved.
5. Allow the tea to cool to room temperature, then refrigerate until chilled.
6. Garnish with lemon slices and serve beside ice cubes.

Portion Size: 1 serving

Preparation Time: 15 minutes (plus chilling time)

Nutritional Information (per serving):

- Calories: 10
- Protein: 0g
- Fat: 0g
- Carbohydrates: 3g
- Fiber: 0g

Lemon Basil Infused Water:

Ingredients:

- 1 lemon, thinly sliced
- 1 handful fresh basil leaves
- 4 cups filtered water
- Ice cubes (optional)

Preparation:

1. In a large pitcher, combine lemon slices and basil leaves.
2. Add filtered water and stir gently to mix.
3. Refrigerate for at least 1 hour to allow flavors to infuse.
4. Serve chilled over ice cubes if desired.

Portion Size: 1 serving

Preparation Time: 5 minutes (plus chilling time)

Nutritional Information (per serving):

- Calories: 0
- Protein: 0g
- Fat: 0g
- Carbohydrates: 0g
- Fiber: 0g

Minty Green Tea Cooler:

Ingredients:

- 2 green tea bags
- 4 cups boiling water
- 1/4 cup fresh mint leaves
- 1 tablespoon raw honey (optional)
- Lemon slices for garnish

Preparation:

1. Place green tea bags and fresh mint leaves in a heatproof pitcher.
2. Pour boiling water over the tea bags and mint leaves, then steep for 5-10 minutes.
3. Remove the tea bags and mint leaves, then discard.
4. Optionally, add raw honey for sweetness and stir until dissolved.
5. Allow the tea to cool to room temperature, then refrigerate until chilled.
6. Serve over ice cubes and garnish with lemon slices.

Portion Size: 1 serving

Preparation Time: 15 minutes (plus chilling time)

Nutritional Information (per serving):

- Calories: 10
- Protein: 0g
- Fat: 0g
- Carbohydrates: 3g
- Fiber: 0g

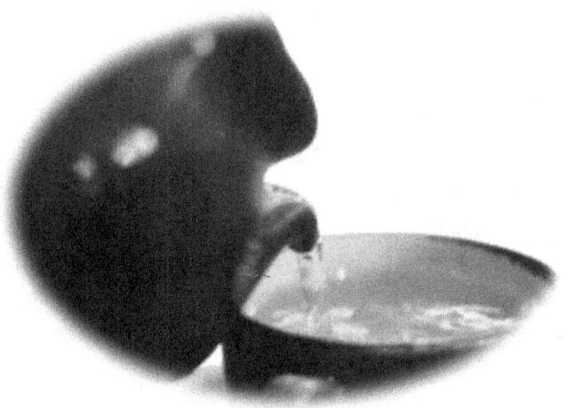

7-DAY MEAL PLAN

DAY 1

BREAKFAST: **Coconut Flour Pancakes**

LUNCH: **Quinoa and Veggie Buddha Bowl**

DINNER: **Lemon Garlic Baked Salmon**

DAY 2

BREAKFAST: **Greek Yogurt Parfait**

LUNCH: **Zucchini Noodles with Avocado Pesto**

DINNER: **Cauliflower Rice Stir-Fry**

DAY 3

BREAKFAST: **Veggie Omelette**

LUNCH: **Salmon Salad with Lemon Dill Dressing**

DINNER: **Baked Chicken with Roasted Vegetables**

DAY 4

BREAKFAST: **Almond Flour Muffins**

LUNCH: **Cauliflower Fried Rice**

DINNER: **Turkey and Vegetable Stuffed Bell Peppers**

DAY 5

BREAKFAST: **Green Smoothie Bowl**

LUNCH: **Lentil and Vegetable Soup**

DINNER: **Lentil and Vegetable Curry**

DAY 6

BREAKFAST: Quinoa Breakfast Bowl

LUNCH: Turkey and Avocado Wrap

DINNER: Grilled Lemon Herb Chicken with Roasted Asparagus

DAY 7

BREAKFAST: Baked Sweet Potato Breakfast Hash

LUNCH: Chickpea and Vegetable Stir-Fry

DINNER: Eggplant and Zucchini Lasagna

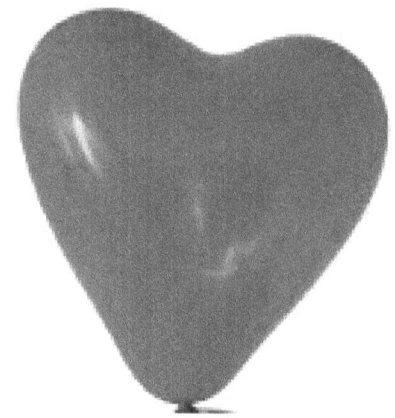

CONCLUSION

Embarking on a journey to combat candida overgrowth and restore balance to your body through dietary changes is a significant step towards reclaiming your health and vitality. Throughout this book, we've delved into the intricacies of candida overgrowth, its signs and symptoms, causes, and preventive measures. We've explored the fundamentals of the candida diet, learning about the foods to avoid and those to embrace to support our body's natural healing processes.

Moreover, we've provided a comprehensive list of candida-friendly recipes, from nourishing breakfast options to satisfying lunch and dinner dishes, as well as refreshing beverages to enjoy throughout the day. These recipes are not only delicious but also crafted with ingredients specifically chosen to aid in the fight against candida overgrowth, providing essential nutrients and promoting overall well-being.

As you incorporate these recipes into your daily routine, remember that healing is a journey, and progress may take time.

Be patient with yourself, listen to your body, and celebrate the small victories along the way. With dedication, perseverance, and a commitment to nourishing your body with wholesome, candida-friendly foods, you can take control of your health and thrive.

Let this book serve as a guide and a source of inspiration as you embark on your candida-fighting journey. May it empower you to make informed choices, embrace a healthier lifestyle, and ultimately achieve a state of balance and wellness.

Here's to your health, happiness, and vitality!

WEEKLY MEAL PLANNER

WEEK _____   MONTH _____

MONDAY

SATURDAY

TUESDAY

SUNDAY

WEDNESDAY

SHOPPING LIST

- ○ _____
- ○ _____
- ○ _____
- ○ _____
- ○ _____
- ○ _____
- ○ _____
- ○ _____

THURSDAY

FRIDAY

NOTES:

- ○ _____
- ○ _____
- ○ _____
- ○ _____

WEEKLY MEAL PLANNER

WEEK ———————————   MONTH ———————————

MONDAY

SATURDAY

TUESDAY

SUNDAY

WEDNESDAY

SHOPPING LIST

- ○ _____
- ○ _____
- ○ _____
- ○ _____
- ○ _____
- ○ _____
- ○ _____
- ○ _____

THURSDAY

FRIDAY

NOTES:

- ○ _____
- ○ _____
- ○ _____
- ○ _____

WEEKLY
MEAL PLANNER

WEEK —————————— MONTH ——————————

MONDAY

SATURDAY

TUESDAY

SUNDAY

WEDNESDAY

SHOPPING LIST

- ○ —————————————
- ○ —————————————
- ○ —————————————
- ○ —————————————
- ○ —————————————
- ○ —————————————
- ○ —————————————
- ○ —————————————

THURSDAY

FRIDAY

NOTES:

- ○ —————————————
- ○ —————————————
- ○ —————————————
- ○ —————————————

WEEKLY MEAL PLANNER

WEEK _____   MONTH _____

MONDAY

SATURDAY

TUESDAY

SUNDAY

WEDNESDAY

SHOPPING LIST

- _____
- _____
- _____
- _____
- _____
- _____
- _____
- _____

THURSDAY

FRIDAY

NOTES:

- _____
- _____
- _____
- _____

WEEKLY
MEAL PLANNER

WEEK —————————— MONTH ——————————

MONDAY

SATURDAY

TUESDAY

SUNDAY

WEDNESDAY

SHOPPING LIST

- O ——————————
- O ——————————
- O ——————————
- O ——————————
- O ——————————
- O ——————————
- O ——————————
- O ——————————

THURSDAY

FRIDAY

NOTES:

- O ——————————
- O ——————————
- O ——————————
- O ——————————

WEEKLY MEAL PLANNER

WEEK ——————————   MONTH ——————————

MONDAY

SATURDAY

TUESDAY

SUNDAY

WEDNESDAY

SHOPPING LIST

- ○ ——————————
- ○ ——————————
- ○ ——————————
- ○ ——————————
- ○ ——————————
- ○ ——————————
- ○ ——————————
- ○ ——————————

THURSDAY

FRIDAY

NOTES:

- ○ ——————————
- ○ ——————————
- ○ ——————————
- ○ ——————————

WEEKLY
MEAL PLANNER

WEEK ——————————— MONTH ———————————

MONDAY

SATURDAY

TUESDAY

SUNDAY

WEDNESDAY

SHOPPING LIST
- ○ _____
- ○ _____
- ○ _____
- ○ _____

THURSDAY
- ○ _____
- ○ _____
- ○ _____
- ○ _____

FRIDAY

NOTES:
- ○ _____
- ○ _____
- ○ _____
- ○ _____

WEEKLY
MEAL PLANNER

WEEK _____   MONTH _____

MONDAY

SATURDAY

TUESDAY

SUNDAY

WEDNESDAY

SHOPPING LIST

- ○ _____
- ○ _____
- ○ _____
- ○ _____

THURSDAY

- ○ _____
- ○ _____
- ○ _____
- ○ _____

FRIDAY

NOTES:

- ○ _____
- ○ _____
- ○ _____
- ○ _____

WEEKLY MEAL PLANNER

WEEK _____   MONTH _____

MONDAY

SATURDAY

TUESDAY

SUNDAY

WEDNESDAY

SHOPPING LIST

- ○ _____
- ○ _____
- ○ _____
- ○ _____
- ○ _____
- ○ _____
- ○ _____
- ○ _____

THURSDAY

FRIDAY

NOTES:

- ○ _____
- ○ _____
- ○ _____
- ○ _____

WEEKLY MEAL PLANNER

WEEK _____   MONTH _____

MONDAY

SATURDAY

TUESDAY

SUNDAY

WEDNESDAY

SHOPPING LIST

- ○ _____
- ○ _____
- ○ _____
- ○ _____
- ○ _____
- ○ _____
- ○ _____
- ○ _____

THURSDAY

FRIDAY

NOTES:

- ○ _____
- ○ _____
- ○ _____
- ○ _____

WEEKLY MEAL PLANNER

WEEK _____   MONTH _____

MONDAY

SATURDAY

TUESDAY

SUNDAY

WEDNESDAY

SHOPPING LIST

- ○ _____
- ○ _____
- ○ _____
- ○ _____

THURSDAY

- ○ _____
- ○ _____
- ○ _____
- ○ _____

FRIDAY

NOTES:

- ○ _____
- ○ _____
- ○ _____
- ○ _____

WEEKLY MEAL PLANNER

WEEK ——————————— MONTH ———————————

MONDAY

SATURDAY

TUESDAY

SUNDAY

WEDNESDAY

SHOPPING LIST

- ○ _____
- ○ _____
- ○ _____
- ○ _____
- ○ _____
- ○ _____
- ○ _____
- ○ _____

THURSDAY

NOTES:
- ○ _____
- ○ _____
- ○ _____

FRIDAY